Beautiful Scars of Hope Workbook

Workbook Companion to Beautiful Scars of Hope

Roxanne Holt and Clint Crawford

Introduction

Clint and I collaborated to create this workbook to help in both independent self-work and reflection or in a treatment setting. This workbook breaks down Beautiful Scars of Hope, the change in thinking throughout my journey and helps relate it to your personal recovery journey. In each chapter of my book you can look at examples of my thinking in active addiction and how I started to change my thinking. As Clint always says, "It's not using and drinking that get us to where we are, it's our thinking."

Individually as you read through you can process your own thoughts and journey with the guided questions we created that Clint has found to be effective in therapeutic settings for years in leading to self-discovery and it will assist you to create action items for change. Ideally, in an independent study environment I would see this workbook being beneficial as a companion to step work to process with a sponsor, or possibly an addition to a women's book study or group.

This workbook can also be helpful used the same way in a treatment setting, group work, outpatient groups or even individually with a therapist. This will help approach treatment in a more specialized way to address challenges in recovery specific to women in recovery. Although addiction is addiction, the truth is that there are challenges and differences that women face in sobriety…..especially in parenting, trauma, relationships, sober sex, self-validation and learning how to love ourselves!

This workbook can be leveraged and useful in many ways. Our goal was to create a companion to my book Beautiful Scars of Hope that takes an honest look at things that aren't talked about openly enough in early recovery, however have a large impact on recovery for women. To provide therapeutic insight from Clint's years of experience working with and treating women in recovery and benefit women in taking an honest look at their stories, their insane thinking and how to take action towards change.

If you are reading this and ready to make a change, I challenge you to identify rather than compare. Many times, when reflecting it is natural to look at the differences to avoid accepting our reality and where we are in our addiction. Instead, look at the similarities, in how our thinking becomes, in the feelings we experience and how our lives and relationships become affected. Although the detail varies from story to story the outcomes and affects of addiction are most often very similar. So, get honest with yourself and take a step towards positive change. As I was once told, you have to go through it to get to the other side…..and although you have to look back, don't stare – learn from it and move forward. This workbook is designed to help you reflect, learn and move forward!

Section One

Reflection Questions About Your Early Childhood and Using

In chapter one Roxanne discusses her early years and also her early using. When talking with patients I often discuss the fact that one's using and drinking is not the core problem. The core problem is found in one's thinking. One finds over, and over again when dealing with addiction, that until a person is able to change the way he/she thinks about addiction he/she will never be able to find sobriety. There are many theories about addiction and what causes it. The reality is whether it is a disease, a behavioral problem, a moral problem, or whatever, at this point, you have a very serious problem and that is where we want to focus. Acknowledging I have a problem at this point, what am I prepared to do about it? It begins with taking a very intense life inventory, starting at the beginning, and walking one's way through every life detail from the past to present.

Some of the things you will have to look at will be uncomfortable. Some of the things from the past you may want to avoid discussing. However, this is where a change in one's thinking becomes so important. Do you truly want to stop using/drinking? If so, you must be willing to be uncomfortable. How you have been thinking up until now has not worked, correct? Then be willing to try looking at things differently for a change, underneath a new light, from a different perspective. It might surprise you at what you discover about yourself. So, let us begin a new journey today.

Section One Questions

1. Did you find any similarities between your early childhood and Roxanne's? If so, what were they? Were there differences? If so, what were they. When working on this question I encourage you to take Roxanne's advice in her introduction. Identify, rather than compare. Many times people struggling with addiction are apt to simply compare, as a way to get out of looking at themselves. For example, "Well, Roxanne had brothers and I was an only child, so this book probably won't help me". Simply relate to her thinking, lack of coping skills, influences, etc. Most of the time people find many similarities between their story and others solely based on how other addicts think and feel regardless of different details.

    _____

    _____

    _____

    _____

    _____

2. Roxanne discussed that early in childhood, her father instilled in her, to "put your big girl britches on, and deal with it". She also discussed that her mother instilled in her to never, "air your dirty laundry". These are ways of thinking, that simply mean, "get over it and move forward", and "don't discuss personal issues with anyone", and can lead to one's not talking about his/her problems, also known as, "stuffing". You will find later in Roxanne's story, that this way of thinking

hindered her ability to get clean and sober in many ways. What ways of thinking did you develop early on in life, that continue to influence your decisions, for which you may see you will need to change moving forward?

_____

_____

_____

_____

_____

3. What person or persons in your early life influenced you the most, whether positively, or negatively. Are they still a part of your life? What kind of relationship do you have with them at this point? Has your using affected those relationships?

_____

_____

_____

_____

_____

4. When did you first try using drugs/alcohol? Where were you? Who were you with? What were your thoughts and feelings about it?

_____

_____

5. At what point in your life, did you realize that perhaps you used more than others, or had a higher tolerance than others?

6. Was there a point where you realized, or at least considered the fact, that you might have a problem with drugs/alcohol? When was this?

7. You heard Roxanne discuss the fact that she turned down several scholarships due to the fact that it would hinder her partying and ability to use at will? At what point did you realize your using was beginning to dictate your decision-making process?

8. Looking back, do you see a point in your life where you found you were trying to convince yourself that you didn't have a problem with drugs/alcohol?

9. Was there anyone in your life who tried to talk to you about your using during this early period? If so, what was your reaction to them? Why do you think they felt the need to try and talk to you about it?

10. You heard Roxanne discuss the fact that in college her grades began to slip, and she began to miss classes. She also discussed that she began having relationship problems with both female friends, and in her dating relationships with males. Looking back, can you pinpoint the time at which your using began to impede on your daily life, and relationships? In what ways? Be specific.

_____
_____
_____
_____
_____

11. We as people develop many of our coping strategies early on in childhood, adolescence, and early adulthood. Looking back was there a point at which your using/drinking became your way of coping with negative thoughts, emotions, and difficult circumstances?

_____
_____
_____
_____
_____

12. Can you at this point, after answering the previous questions, identify any ways in which your thinking promoted your continued use of drugs/alcohol?

Additional Workspace if Needed:

Section Two

Identifying Denial and Delusion

As I said earlier, one's thinking must change in order for one to find sobriety. When looking at the many ways one's thinking about their addiction can be misguided, the biggest issue comes in the form of denial and delusion. An important fact to remember is most of the time, if not always, you will see denial, or at least forms of denial first, then as one's addiction progresses, you will see this denial turn into complete delusion. Many people often think of denial as being very overt in nature. Such as, "I don't have a problem, and I can stop using any time I want!" This is a form of denial, of course, however the biggest form of denial, which is the hardest to deal with as a therapist, is covert denial.

Covert denial can come in many forms. For example, "Well yeah, I drink a little too much at times, but I still have all my bills paid and I go to work every day, so what is the problem?" You can also see covert denial in this argument, "Well pills are my real problem, so I'll just quit using pills and just drink......I have never had a problem with drinking." Further, you can see covert denial in this statement, "Well yeah I use, but if you had been through what I have been through, you would have to use too!" There are hundreds of examples one could use here, perhaps you are now thinking of ways in which you have done this or may be doing it now. One rule of thumb to look for in finding whether or not your thinking is flawed is to ask yourself, "Am I rationalizing, justifying, or minimizing my using in any way?"

As I stated, at some point in addiction, denial becomes complete delusion. Roxanne discusses the fact that her father once confronted her about the fact that he had found 15 liquor bottles stuffed in various places of her couch. Her reply, "Yeah but they are JUST pints!" Her thinking had become completely delusional at this point. In her mind she truly could not see how serious her situation was. Denial and delusion are a flawed, and dangerous coping mechanism which is fueled by the fear of facing one's truth. Roxanne discusses often with patients she works with, who are in denial, that she understands where they are because she was once there as well. She says, "I knew if I ever admitted I had a problem, then I would have to do something about it, and I didn't want to, because I didn't believe I was capable to stop using at that point in my life." So, in that statement you hear that her denial and delusion was fueled by what? Fear.

In dealing with patients in treatment centers, I love having staff members around who are in recovery. They are proof to patients that recovery is possible, and it helps, and encourages them to face their fears head on, knowing that anyone who gets clean/sober has to do it, but most importantly, that it is possible. So, I challenge you to look at Roxanne's story, and find the hope you need to face your problem, head on, in all of its ugliness, and uncomfortableness, knowing recovery is possible for you, just as it was for Roxanne.

Section Two Questions

Examples of minimizing, justifying, and rationalizing one's using:

Minimizing – "Well I only have two drinks a night", when the reality is the two drinks consisted of two stadium cups full of straight vodka.

Justifying – "If you had been through what I have been through you would use too", when the reality is every human being on earth goes through hard times, and there is always someone who has had it if not the same as you, then even worse. This also includes people in recovery who had very hard times after getting clean/sober who still did not return to using.

Rationalizing – "Well yeah, I drink a lot but I have never had a DUI or been locked up, so I must not have a problem", when the reality is your relationships and health are a wreck and everyone in your life realizes you have a problem but you.

1. Can you identify any ways in which you have exhibited, or are currently exhibiting traits of denial in your thinking regarding your addiction? Be specific.

_____

_____

_____

2. What explanations would you offer to me, if I asked you to prove to me you are not an addict or alcoholic? Perhaps others have attempted to talk to you about your using in the past. What did you say to them? Did you make any excuses for your using? Did your offer any arguments to them about why they were wrong? What were they?

3. In reading Roxanne's story, what forms of denial did you see her exhibit when confronted about her own addiction.

4. Think of other ways one can exhibit denial besides the ones mentioned and write them down.

5. Are you afraid of looking at your past, and things you have done in active addiction? What scares you the most and why?

6. Many times we hear people say, "You have to get honest". While this is true, I think there needs to be more specificity to this statement. Yes, one needs to get honest, not just with others, but with themselves. Many times a person struggling with addiction has told themselves many things before they ever offer excuses to other people. So, considering this, in what ways have you minimized, rationalized, or justified your using in your head once the thoughts that you may have a problem have crept into your mind?

_____

_____

_____

_____

7. Does the fact that others, like Roxanne, have found sobriety give you hope that you can too? If not, why not? What makes it different for you? Do you think it will be harder for you to get clean than someone else? Why?

_____

_____

_____

_____

_____

Additional Workspace if Needed:

_____

_____

_____

_____

_____

Section Three

Breaking Through Denial and Accepting My Reality

Have you ever tried to tell a delusional person that they are delusional? If so, how'd that work out for you? It doesn't work…..because they are still delusional. That is much of what early recovery and treatment is – breaking through denial and delusion to see and accept our realities. Throughout my story you read several examples of denial, as well as full blown delusion. Deep down I knew if I accepted my reality, I would then HAVE to do something about it. I was so full of fear….fear of failure, fear of facing consequences of my actions, etc., that I allowed denial and delusion to comfort me as a defense mechanism, because I was too afraid to accept my reality……and I could not maintain any length of sobriety until I became willing to do so.

I talked about it in my book, about arriving at treatment the last time and remembering the moment reality came rushing in and slapped me in the face. I remember I was sitting outside by myself and had been there in treatment about two or two and half weeks and it hit me. "Look at yourself Roxanne." "How has this become my reality?" "You're dying". "You're so afraid to live you've abandoned your kids when they needed you the most!" As my thinking started to clear I could think through the denial and acknowledge that…"You're not a victim, you're a survivor and too afraid to live and face life". "You're not 'heroin chic', you're almost dead from malnutrition and drug abuse". "You're not a good mother….yes, you're willing to die for them…but what about living for them? What about being present in their lives?" and so much more.

Outside of the fear that facing my reality meant I had to change, I was terrified that I couldn't maintain life and sobriety successfully. I mean I had never been able to in the past, right? I was also fearful of being honest and facing my reality because I think a part of me thought if I ever allowed myself to fully feel everything I had been running from for so long, I couldn't handle it and it would break me. There's an obvious example of denial and delusion right there….using and drinking had broken me long before I accepted my reality, so what was I really afraid of? Part of changing my thinking and breaking through the denial was to face things honestly. Let's face it, I was already hurting myself and everyone I loved worse by using, than facing my reality could ever hurt….regardless of anyone else, I had to finally become willing to be honest with myself.

Section Three Questions

1. How has your using affected your health?

2. How has your using affected your finances?

3. How has your using affected you legally? How could it have affected you legally if you were held accountable? (If you have no legal consequences skip to the next question).

4. If you have children, how has your using affected your relationship with them? How has your using affected them personally? Where are they currently living? Have other people in your life had to step in to take care of them or help you take care of them, such as your parents or children's services? If you are in a situation where someone else is currently taking care of them, are they doing better under their care, (sleeping better, improved eating, improved grades, etc.) (If you do not have children skip to the next question).

_____

_____

_____

_____

5. Has your using affected your career or education? In what ways?

_____

_____

_____

_____

6. How has your using affected other relationships you have such as parents, spouse, siblings, friends, partner?

7. How has your using affected you mentally?

8. How has your using influenced your own idea of self-worth and self-value?

9. How would your relationships, health, career, and overall well-being be affected if you were to stop using?

10. Do you believe you are worth it? Why or why not?

Additional Workspace if Needed:

Section Four

Trauma and Addiction

The first thing one should realize about trauma is that it is relative to the person. With trauma, just as with addiction, one should seek to identify rather than compare. It is common for people to look and listen to other people's traumatic stories and quickly begin comparing. For example, "Yes, my father was abusive, but at least he never molested me. I'm not even going to talk about mine……..her's is way worse than mine!" On the other hand, another common thing to see happen when people are comparing versus identifying is to judge other people's trauma. For example, "She is actually saying her dog dying was traumatic?......Are you kidding me?" Again, trauma is relative. What might not be considered a big deal for one person, can be very big for another.

Roxanne discusses her own trauma and has shared that for the longest she did not want to talk about her trauma in groups where others were discussing their own, because she felt responsible for what had happened to her in a way. Meaning, she was an adult, and she was in an abusive relationship with a man who was also actively using. So, in her mind she felt like that negated anything that had happened to her. The reality of it all is that trauma is trauma. It affects you mentally and even physically and regardless of how the trauma came to be in one's life, it has a powerful effect on one's outlook, mental stability, and overall health.

What does this mean for an addict? Well, quite simply it means you need to deal with your addiction, but you also must deal with your trauma as well, however, you must realize that they are two separate issues. Why would we say this? It sounds simple enough to state that one has addiction and trauma, and those are obviously two different things, right?   Unfortunately, many times people tend to lump the two together into one big problem and view it that way. For example, "Well, I started using because it helped me escape from my thoughts and feelings about being raped. Since I can't go back in time and change the fact that I was raped, I won't be able to quit using either, because that is the only way I can deal with it!" So essentially, the two problems feed each other. The negative thoughts and feelings from the trauma fuel the desire for continued use, and because when one is using they are not affectively coping with the trauma, it remains unaddressed and therefore is never effectively dealt with.

The reality for a person who has both addiction and trauma issues, is that both must be dealt with. If one only addresses his/her addiction, yet never talks about or addresses the trauma, he/she will not be able to remain clean as the negative thoughts and feelings will eventually become too much. There is an old saying that explains this perfectly,….."Our secrets keep us sick". If one only addresses the trauma yet never addresses his/her addiction, he/she will never remain clean, as without adequately learning how to live clean and sober, one will always return to using.

This is where the hard work comes in. Just as the fear of facing one's addiction leads to denial, the fear of facing one's trauma leads to avoidant behaviors. In some cases, there is a form of denial that says, "It wasn't that bad, I mean I got over it". In Roxanne's case there was a certain denial which said, "Well I was grown and actively using, in a relationship with a guy who was also using, so really…….I asked for it. I have no right to complain…..I mean there are people who had horrible things happen to them when they were kids and had no control over it." In doing this, she essentially negated the affect her trauma had on her life and for a long time it hindered her ability to effectively deal with it.

Another old saying is, "Name the dragon, and you take its power". When it comes to trauma, and effectively dealing with it, one must start with acknowledging the affect it had on you. Notice I didn't say simply, "acknowledge the trauma". Why? Because there are many people (Roxanne was one), who will in fact say things such as, "I was raped", yet never go into any detail about it whatsoever. Or, to use Roxanne again, "My husband died", yet for the longest she would never discuss how that affected her. She wouldn't discuss for instance how she sat up all night after her husband had died, wondering how she would ever tell her boys once they awoke the next morning their father was dead. She wouldn't discuss the details of her trauma. For example, she wouldn't discuss what it was like to be held down, raped, and burned with cigarettes to the point that her body still holds the scars.

Roxanne will tell you today, that once she got to the point where she fully faced her dragon, and named it, in every detail, in all its ugliness, she immediately began healing. Was it over night? Of course not. However, it was a start. A place from which she could get a foothold and move forward. Yet, it began with that first step of naming the dragon. Today Roxanne has her power back. She can openly talk about her trauma. Does it still bother her at times? Of course, it does. However, is she consumed by it today? Absolutely not! It can be the same for you………..if you are willing to name your dragon.

Section Four Questions

1. What traumatic experience or experiences have you had in your life? How old were you?

2. Have you ever talked about your trauma to anyone else when you were not high or drunk? If so, did it help?

3. What scares or bothers you the most about discussing your past trauma?

4. What thoughts and feelings do you have when you think about your trauma?

   _____

   _____

   _____

   _____

5. Do you have nightmares or panic attacks related to your past trauma? What feelings do you have associated with this (anger, sadness, fear, etc.)?

   _____

   _____

   _____

   _____

6. Do you feel that the fact your past trauma happened was your fault, or in part, your fault? If so, why?

   _____

   _____

   _____

   _____

7. Do you blame someone for not intervening, or protecting you?

8. Does your past trauma cause you problems with trusting people today?

9. What ways does your past trauma affect your present-day life? For example, are you hyper-vigilant, do you become uncomfortable when someone is behind you, do you startle easily, do you have problems being intimate with the opposite sex?

10. Have you ever had the feeling that you are broken or dirty? Why?

11. How often do you think about your past trauma?

12. Do certain situations or people cause you to think about your past trauma more? Why?

Additional Workspace if Needed:

Section Five

Spiritual Development in Recovery

Throughout my journey in recovery I have also been on a journey with my spirituality. Although I am flawed at best, spirituality is something I continuously work on, and strive to improve on daily. As long as I remain humble and teachable, I stay in a place where I can grow spiritually. In my book, I described having a relationship with God, and throughout my story as something I never thought I needed. Today however, I know I would not be sober or be who I am today without my personal relationship with God. I struggled during this transition. I remember getting to a point of acceptance about my addiction and being told that I would have to rely on a power greater than myself to treat it and thinking, "Well now what? I can't continue to use, but the only solution is something I don't believe in or participate in....religion." But I was wrong, it not about religion, it's about spiritual growth and development. I remember hearing someone say once that, "Religion is for people that don't want to go to Hell, but spirituality is for people who have already been".

When choosing to live a life of recovery you are challenged to ACTIVELY apply spiritual principles in your everyday life and in all that you think, do and say. Simply put, spiritual principles are a good and honest way to live, and if you are consciously working to apply them in all that you do, your new way of living cannot co-exist with the behaviors that accompany active addiction and alcoholism. Having knowledge of something and being able to acknowledge it in your actions and life are two different things. In my book, I talked about knowing how to get sober but not knowing how to stay sober. Similarly, when looking at what is "right and wrong" in my behavior, I had a knowledge of what "right" was, but I wasn't acknowledging that within my own behavior and actively implementing that knowledge in my everyday actions. Having knowledge of recovery and living a life of recovery are very different things. Faith without works is dead….. knowing isn't enough, you must put action to it! Just like with anything you are asked to do or is suggested to you when begin your journey, spirituality is no different, you just have to start with remaining OPEN and WILLING….and you will be amazed at how your concept of spirituality and how your personal growth in your faith will develop and change along the way.

In my book I shared about avoiding a connection with God or any concept loosely even related, because I was embarrassed at how uneducated I was about the subject, I was mad at life and the circumstances I had along the way and I was full of FEAR. However, when I sat still long enough to pay attention to the people around me that God was placing in my life, and honestly just became willing to get out of my own way, I finally had relief. I didn't have to fight everything and everyone anymore, I didn't have to manipulate or attempt to control, I didn't have to validate or search for acceptance…..I had a choice and a freedom like I have never experienced….and I just had to be honest. In touching on and speaking about spirituality everyone is different and it becomes very personal, so I again remind you to challenge yourself to honestly answer the questions and reflect on your thinking. Identify rather than compare, and remain open to thinking differently to gain a different outcome.

In the past, I would walk into a church or meeting and easily look for or point out people I perceived as "hypocrites" to prove to myself why the concept of spirituality would not work for me. Much like every other aspect of my recovery I had to change my thinking. I shifted my perspective to look at how it can and does help me in my life and in my recovery, and seek the people I find hope in. After I stopped drinking and using, my thinking did not change overnight. I would walk into a room and subconsciously would immediately start to observe and "size people up" so to speak. My motives were typically selfish in nature, "Who could I manipulate if I needed to?", "Who should I make friends with to benefit me in some way?", "Is there anyone who I should be afraid of?", etc. My thinking has changed today, I changed spiritually therefore, when walking in a room I have genuine motives and do not immediately start to evaluate those around me in judgement, rather I look for what I can contribute, now my subconscious looks for opportunities to add to someone's day rather than self-serving motives. In recovery I get out what I am willing to put in, are you willing to identify and be genuine in your effort to grow spiritually?

Many people ask me what I do to maintain and grow spiritually. I complete readings geared to help me maintain a focus on spiritual growth and continued development daily. I pray to talk to God (throughout the day), meditate to find peace, quiet my mind and listen to Him for guidance and I read my Bible, Recovery Bible and other literature to continue learning about Him. I ask for guidance every morning and thank Him every night before I go to sleep….this is what works for me. It may be different for you, but you won't know until you are willing to explore and challenge yourself. Let's remember, if you are in active addiction or newly sober you can usually acknowledge your way isn't working anymore AND if you are comfortable early on, you are not growing – I encourage you to stay teachable and to try something different.

Section Five Questions

1. As of now, what is your concept of God, spirituality, and/or religion?

2. Do you consider yourself a believer in God? An Atheist (one who does not believe there is any God or higher being/beings)? An Agnostic (one who believes there is some form or type of higher being, but do not identify it/him/her with any certain name?

3. At what point or age did you consider yourself a believer, atheist, agnostic? Was there anything in your life that happened to cause you to change your belief system? If so, what was it?

4. Have you had any negative experiences in the past with religion (churches, church people, pastors, "Christians", etc.) If so, describe. (If not skip ahead to the next question).

5. If you were or are a believer in God, in your current situation do you feel angry or distant from God? If so, why? If you feel distant from God, do you feel it will be hard to become close to God again? Why? Do you feel worthy of forgiveness or love? (If you do not have a belief in God, skip forward to the next question).

6. Do you believe in evil? If so, do you believe there is also an opposing force (good)? Let's say you and I are having a discussion about this. Convince there is evil in the world. Convince me there is good in the world. What evidence can you give me for both?

_____

_____

_____

_____

_____

7. Can you think of a time or place in your life where you feel or have felt completely at peace? Describe it. What elements of that place and/or time made you feel that way?

_____

_____

_____

_____

_____

8. If you do not subscribe to any God, spirituality, or religion, does the concept of finding a higher power make you feel hopeless to overcome your addiction? Why?

9. Do you have any feelings of anger, resentment, shame, or aggravation, when someone says you need to go to church, pray, or find God? Why?

10. What spiritual principles (honesty, humility, compassion, etc) do you feel are lacking in your life? Describe. What can you do differently to begin implanting those in your everyday life?

11. Do you blame God, or some higher being, or fate, for past situations which have happened in your life? Describe why and name specific situations.

_____

_____

_____

_____

_____

12. Do you have a concept of, "God's Will", for your life? If so, describe it. Or, do you believe God has a certain plan, path, or purpose for your life? If so, what is it? Perhaps you believe this, however at the moment you are not certain what it is. If so, discuss any thoughts you may have as to what God's plan, path, or purpose for you could possibly be?

_____

_____

_____

_____

_____

Additional Workspace if Needed:

Section Six

Self-Love and Self-Worth

There is a common characteristic, I have found in my experience of working in the addiction field over the years that seems to be, for addicts in active addiction, and in early recovery, a sub-conscious occurrence, but one that many do. They have a habit of never looking themselves directly in the eye when they look into a mirror. They may brush their hair, wash their face, brush their teeth……but they avoid looking themselves directly in the eye. Like the book, The Picture of Dorian Gray, Dorian cannot look upon his own portrait, or he will surely be destroyed, as his portrait revealed his true self, including all his past mis-deeds and sins…….so it was kept in a room, wrapped in paper, so he never had to face it.

Why is this so common in addicts in active addiction and early recovery? I believe there are a number of reasons. Guilt, shame, regret, self-resentment, self-loathing,…..and on and on. I have lost count of how many addicts have told me over the years, "Clint I hate myself!". "I hate what I have done, and the kind of person I am!". Have you ever stared directly into your own eyes in a mirror? Try it sometime. You will find, that it can be intensely intimate. It is, in a way, like looking into your own soul. Why do you think for many people, especially addicts, this is hard to do? I think that it is again, much like Dorian Gray and his portrait, simply too overwhelming.

You may currently be in this place. You may have no sense of self-love or self-worth left. I can tell you this is a normal feeling for addicts in active addiction and in early recovery. This also brings an importance of mentioning shame and guilt in early recovery. They are similar in meaning but also different. Guilt can be likened to, "Oh my God, what have I done?" Shame can be likened to, "Oh my God, what have I become?" There is often, for addicts, intense shame. I have become someone I never dreamed I would be……..someone who does (or has done) awful things! What is wrong with me? I hate myself! I'm a worthless human being!!!! Again, all very normal feelings that addicts go through. In Roxanne's story she discusses this and the rush of feelings she felt when it finally hit her about two weeks into treatment.

The key is to remember, you are lovable, and you have true worth. The fact alone that you are a living, breathing, human being holds value in itself. It means you have a chance to change it all. You have a chance, right here, right now, to turn it all around. I often deal with patients who are very busy beating themselves up over their past. One thing I tell them repeatedly is this, "Okay, so you made a mess of things, you did things you wish you hadn't done, you hurt people, you hurt yourself…….okay, I'll give you that…..that is sad and a shame. But, you know what would really be sad, and a crying shame? If you were still out there somewhere using….still living the same way, doing the same things….but today, you are here, trying to get clean and sober, and today……you are not the person you were then!

Right now you are all down and out over who you WERE then, and I'm standing here telling you I am proud of who you ARE right now!'

Again, you deserve love, and you are worthy! Worthy of love and happiness and peace of mind. However, you have to make some very real changes. Changes that will be tough and uncomfortable. Yet, I promise it is worth it! Roxanne often tells people in treatment and very early recovery, "If I could just grab you and shake you, and let you feel how good a life in recovery can be, you would never want to go back and use again!" So, today, begin by forgiving yourself. Whatever you have done in the past, whatever you have been……forgive yourself. That doesn't mean elements of your past actions may not hang around for a while, or that consequences won't show up at times, but I promise it will get better with time. The reality of Dorian Gray…….had he been willing to look at himself, and how he was living his life early on……he could have changed everything…..and learned to love himself.

Section Six Questions

1. Do you love yourself? Why or why not? If not, how can you begin to love yourself more? How will you measure it?

2. If I asked you, on a scale of 1 to 10, where you would rate your level of self-love, what would you say? Why

3. Do you feel worthy enough to be loved or cared for by others? Why or why not?

4. If you answered, "No", to question 3, I want you to convince me with your best argument/arguments, of why you are not worthy of love or the care of others.

_____
_____
_____
_____
_____

5. Is there someone in your life, who has made past mistakes, or perhaps hurt you, or both, yet, you still love them and care for them? If so, why do you still love them and care for them? How could your argument for why you still love and care for that person be applied to your feelings of being unlovable or unworthy of the care of others if you feel you are unlovable and unworthy?

_____
_____
_____
_____
_____

6. What do you need to forgive yourself for? How can you begin to forgive yourself?

_____
_____
_____

7. Do you feel worthy of forgiveness? Why or why not?

8. Have you forgiven others before for things they have done? If so, why did you forgive them? If you have forgiven someone for something in the past, yet feel you are not worthy of forgiveness, explain your thinking in a paragraph as to what the difference is?

9. Describe what self-worth means to you. Is it based on what you have (money, clothes, etc.), or is it something more? What is that, "something more"? How can you begin to build up your sense of self-worth?

10. Describe what self-love means to you. Does it have to do more with self-pride, talents, looks, or is it something more? What is that "something more"?

11. If I asked your parents, children, spouse, significant other, why they love you, what answer/answers do you think they would give me and why?

12. Think about this statement: Self-worth is not based on how others view me, but how I view me. What does that statement mean to you personally? How do you

currently view yourself? If you are not currently happy with who you are at the moment, describe who you would like to be, or the type of person you would like to be? How can you begin to become that person?

_____

_____

_____

_____

_____

_____

Additional Workspace if Needed:

_____

_____

_____

_____

_____

_____

_____

_____

Section Seven

Relationships Part One

One of the biggest challenges for a woman dealing with addiction and also in sobriety, revolves around relationships. Whether it involves currently being in an unhealthy relationship, rebuilding relationships that have been harmed or even destroyed due to addiction, or new relationships in sobriety, a great deal of attention and effort must be directed here. You read in Roxanne's story of how at different points in her active addiction, and later in sobriety, she dealt with all three of the areas just mentioned. This section will be the first part, of a three-part series. That should show you the importance that relationships play in the life of anyone dealing with addiction, but especially for women. This section will serve as a way to first look at how you currently view and define what a relationship is, and/or how you think a relationship should look.

Section Seven Questions

1. How do you define a healthy relationship? What attributes would you say a healthy relationship has, or should have?

   _____

   _____

   _____

   _____

   _____

2. Can you say, honestly, that you have ever been in a healthy relationship? If yes, describe what makes it healthy. If no, why not?

   _____

   _____

   _____

   _____

3. How do you define an unhealthy relationship? Describe what makes it unhealthy. Have you ever been in, or are you currently in an unhealthy relationship? If yes, describe what makes it unhealthy?

   _____

   _____

   _____

_____

_____

4. How do you define love? In her book, Roxanne discussed the difference between sex and intimacy. In your own words, define the difference between sex and intimacy, and how do you relate to those definitions? Provide examples?

_____

_____

_____

_____

5. Do you have past trauma, either physical, sexual, or emotional? If yes, how does that effect your relationships today, or how has it effected relationships up to this point?

_____

_____

_____

_____

6. Create a list describing all the characteristics of your ideal partner (we will come back to this list in a later section). This does not necessarily mean physical

characteristics. Every woman obviously has an ideal partner in mind in terms of looks. However, this list should focus more on what values they have, what they add to the relationship outside of monetary and material things, how they treat you, etc. In short, what kind of person would your ideal partner be?

_____

_____

_____

_____

7. Are you currently in a relationship with someone who is in active addiction, abusive, or both? Why do you remain in this relationship? Can you honestly say you are happy and fulfilled in this relationship? Why or why not?

_____

_____

_____

_____

8. Are you currently in a relationship with someone you would say is your ideal partner, or at least close to that? How has your addiction affected that relationship? Be specific.

9. How has your addiction affected your ability to pursue a healthy relationship? Be specific.

10. When is the last time you had sex sober? How does the thought of having sex and intimacy sober, make you feel? Be specific?

Additional Workspace if Needed:

Section Eight

Relationships Part Two

Now that you have looked at how you define and view relationships overall, let's look at why. Understanding your motives in your relationships is vital to looking objectively at your part in an unhealthy relationship, but more importantly how to learn to avoid the same mistakes and pitfalls while moving forward in recovery. In my book I discussed looking at my past relationships and what my motives were, in a nutshell what I am looking for out of this relationship and then what am I willing to settle for in a relationship due to my addiction, poor self-esteem and self-worth. Before I was able to learn how to engage in a healthy relationship, I had to take an honest look at why I sought the unhealthy relationships I had in the past. Did they "co-sign" my behavior, did they make me feel safe, were they fun, did they make me feel beautiful or special when I couldn't do that for myself? At some point I can say yes to all of these questions.

When reflecting on your answers from the first section on relationships you looked at unhealthy relationships you have had up to this point. If you are currently in a relationship and using together, what changes are you prepared to make if needed to maintain your sobriety….how willing are you? I discussed a sense of survivor's guilt when getting sober and having to establish boundaries in a codependent relationship, which was difficult initially, but necessary for me to heal and grow in a life of recovery. If you are single, how do you approach building a healthy relationship in the future, what can you learn from your past relationships. Are you allowing your past trauma hold you prisoner from enjoying a happy relationship and intimacy with someone? These are all things you have to be willing to examine and be honest with yourself about when you start to heal, grow and learn to not only get sober but, live a life of recovery and be genuinely happy and fulfilled. A relationship is meant to add to your life and happiness, part of the recovery process is learning what that looks like and how to achieve it. If you can't clearly define what you are looking for and wanting in a relationship and understanding what your part is in that definition, how will you achieve it?

You'll remember when reading my story, I talked about someone once telling me, "You attract what you are putting out". That was a sobering and humbling thought, because it was true. And the more honest I became I was able to see how my standards of what was acceptable and what I deserved in a relationship became more and more unhealthy as my addiction progressed. I felt broken and damaged and couldn't imagine someone loving me that wasn't equally broken and damaged, so they could love me without judging me, but the reality was that was just because I was still judging myself. Yes, I have a past. I am an addict, an alcoholic, a widow, a survivor of physical, mental, emotional and sexual abuse, a single mother, getting sober and starting over…..my first thought was, "Nobody healthy and in their right mind would want to be with me". But I learned how to love and validate myself, look at how I define relationships and what I bring to them, check my motives before reacting, and respect myself BEFORE I was able to be a part of a healthy couple.

I remember being terrified to engage in relationship once I was sober and life started getting better again, almost like I didn't trust myself. I thought a healthy and loving relationship just wasn't going to be in the cards for me, but I was wrong. Remember, if you are too comfortable in your recovery and putting yourself in a box, you aren't growing. Push yourself to examine the uncomfortable parts of your past that you need to in order to move forward and have healthy intimacy in your future. As hard as it was at times and as uncomfortable as it could be facing certain parts of my past, I can tell you it was the best thing I could have done for my future and worth it. I don't believe I could be in a relationship without a relapse before I became willing to take a hard, honest look at how I thought about sex, love, men, validation and my mistakes. Today I am happily engaged and have someone that loves and accepts me seeing beauty and strength in my past…..I'm no longer broken, damaged or held prisoner by my past mistakes and abuser, and you can be happy, sober and fulfilled in a relationship too!

Section Eight Questions

1. Create a list of any significant, romantic relationships up to this point.

    _____

    _____

    _____

    _____

    _____

2. In looking at the list you created, mark which relationships you considered healthy or unhealthy and why. This is where you need to be brutally honest yourself, and objective as possible.

    _____

    _____

    _____

    _____

3. Now look at your list, what were your motives in those relationships? What attracted you to them initially?

    For example, if they didn't have access to drugs and help you continue in your addiction, would you have wanted to be in a relationship with them? Did they help you financially or offer you security or a place to live? Did they make you feel better about yourself? (I shared at one point I would surround myself with people a little "sicker" than I thought I was to feel better about what I was doing). Were you trying to "save" them? Were they a distraction? Were they convenient? Etc., etc., the list goes on and on…..

_____
_____
_____
_____

4. Have you ever had a sexual relationship where drugs and alcohol were not involved? If yes, how was this different? If no, why do you think that is?

_____
_____
_____
_____

5. Let's take a look at your behaviors associated with your sexual relationships in the past. I'll ask you to recall and list examples of when you displayed some behaviors in the past. Please note that I am not asking that you remember or list names and specifics about your past sexual experiences. I am asking that you list examples of when, what and why you were using sex when displaying the below behaviors.

Have you ever used sex to manipulate someone or get something you wanted? If yes, list examples.

Have you ever used sex to validate yourself (need someone to recognize or affirm my opinion or feelings – for example I only believe I am pretty, if you think I am pretty and tell me that). If yes, list examples.

Have you ever used sex to make someone jealous, for attention or for revenge? If yes, list examples.

_____
_____
_____
_____
_____

6. How have your thoughts and behaviors in your sexual relationships caused harm to others? Who have you harmed and how?

_____
_____
_____
_____

7. If you have experienced any type of trauma (emotional, physical, mental or sexual) what impact can you identify it having on your relationships?

_____

_____

_____

_____

_____

8. In the previous section you were asked to explain your understanding of the difference between sex and intimacy. Have you ever experienced an intimate relationship that did not involve sex? If so, describe the dynamics of that relationship.

_____

_____

_____

_____

9. When reflecting on my past sexual experiences and trauma at times I would have feelings of shame, guilt, embarrassment, dirty or less than. When working with other woman I often ask, when you lay down to go to sleep at night….what still eats at you? Typically, the response is similar to the feelings I shared above.

In your past sexual experiences are there things you carry guilt, shame or embarrassment about? If so, what are they? (This again is a time where you have to challenge yourself to be brutally honest, if it still bothers you for any reason it is important to address it).

_____

_____

_____

_____

_____

10. Typically, in early recovery it is suggested that women avoid dating or being in sexual relationships for a period of time in order to address these very questions before clouding our thinking with hormones and heightened emotions. How does the thought of not being engaged in a relationship for awhile make you feel? (Even married couples initially are encouraged to love one another from a distance or get well independent of one another first). Does it cause you any fear or anxiety? If so, why? Be specific in your response.

_____

_____

_____

_____

_____

11. In looking back at your responses, can you identify any patterns or unhealthy behaviors you need to focus on addressing? List fears or challenges you may

have about relationships in sobriety? (Consider your current relationship status when answering this question. However, be honest. I have a friend that was married for over ten years and was terrified to have sex when returning home from treatment, because she was afraid to have sex sober, insecure about her ability to still please him sexually, etc. Even women currently in relationships face similar fears about sex and intimacy when getting clean and sober.

_____

_____

_____

_____

Additional Workspace if Needed:

_____

_____

_____

_____

_____

_____

_____

Section Nine

Relationships Part Three

Now that we have identified and are more aware of the aspects surrounding unhealthy relationships, let us take a look at healthy relationships. In your answers to the questions in the prior sections, by now, hopefully you have become more aware of your personal fears and challenges in relationships, and possibly your past mistakes in how you viewed relationships. We all have an internal need for love, sex, and intimacy. In fact, these are some of the things that can make life so rewarding and fulfilling. Yet, we must be aware at all times that healthy relationships take work and commitment. This holds an even stronger meaning for a person in sobriety, as sometimes the past can cloud up the present, meaning, old feelings and memories as well as shame and guilt can sabotage a current relationship, or keep one from being able to successfully develop a healthy relationship.

Section Nine Questions

1. Now that you are more aware of your fears and challenges regarding relationships, what aspects of your past can you see as possibly having a negative impact on a new or current relationship? For example: issues of trust, constantly expecting the person in a new relationship to hurt you, a fear that a new person will find out about your past actions in active addiction and no longer want to be with you, etc. Be specific.

   _____

   _____

   _____

   _____

2. In active addiction we create a new normal and become comfortable with chaos. It is typical to sabotage or create chaos within relationships out of a fear of the unknown, or failure. This most often is related to simply not fully knowing how to function in a healthy relationship. A typical reaction to this fear is to not communicate, as well as approach the fear of being hurt due to feeling vulnerable in the relationship, with a "get them before they get me", mentality. Since getting sober, can you identify times this has been true in your own behavior? Give examples of how this affected your relationships. What was your partner's reaction?

3. In Roxanne's book she discussed the moment she was told that you attract what you put out. Refer back to the list you made in the first section on relationships, concerning your ideal partner. Of the characteristics and attributes you listed, which of these do you currently possess yourself? Provide examples.

4. Now look at the attributes you do not currently possess. In thinking along the same lines, you cannot possibly expect to receive the benefits of those attributes from a partner, without giving your partner the same in return, again, you attract what you put out. Create a list of ways or actions you can practice incorporating those attributes into your personality. For example: "If I want to find a partner I can trust, I must also be trustworthy". So, how

do I go about becoming trustworthy in my every day life? Do this for each of the attributes you listed. * A typical thing to hear when discussing this topic is, "Well, I'll give respect if they respect me first!" The problem with this is that when a person is actively seeking a partner to share his/her life with, they look for attributes which line up with their own personal values. Therefore, if you do not exhibit those positive values, and are unwilling to practice them from the beginning, it will be hard to ever develop a healthy relationship. Once more, you attract what you are putting out!

_____

_____

_____

_____

_____

5. A common mistake when embarking on a new relationship once in recovery is achieving balance. By maintaining our program of recovery and what made us the person we are today we gain the ability to have healthy relationships. Once in a relationship however, we sacrifice aspects of our program to engage more and spend time with our significant other and lose what they were attracted to in the first place. In Roxanne sharing her experience, once she began a relationship she communicated the importance of her recovery early on and I was supportive of her, however in the past she

struggled with balance in her relationships. So, the question becomes, how can you protect your sobriety and maintain balance between working a program of recovery and being actively engaged in a healthy and fulfilling relationship? Have you been codependent in your past relationships? What checks, and balances can you put into place to help you avoid letting things slip or getting too wrapped up to where your sobriety is put into jeopardy?

_____

_____

_____

_____

6. A common concern for women in recovery getting into relationships is, do I tell them about my past and things that happened in my active addiction. Unfortunately, there isn't a clear-cut answer to this response. How much and what depends on you and the relationship. My question for you is what fears do you have about sharing your past with your new partner? They are fears for a reason. The most important thing to remember here is be willing to have the difficult conversations and discuss comfort levels with one another. The key is to look at what you fear? Feelings of shame, fear of abandonment, etc. Mostly you have to be true to yourself and honest enough to where there are not secrets in the relationship or fears of being found out

later in the relationship. Who you were in active addiction is not who you are today, that is a part of active addiction and does not define you – when you love and accept yourself, these answers become easier and you are able to better define your comfort level in sharing information with your partner

_____

_____

_____

_____

_____.

7. Another concern is, what if my partner is not in recovery and wants to drink around me? Or, what if they are in recovery and relapse? Are you comfortable with establishing healthy boundaries and putting your sobriety first? Boundaries are not threats or stipulations, they are simply clearly communicated lines of respect to protect yourself from sacrificing your sobriety or serenity. If you are not comfortable with this, you are most likely not ready to be in a serious relationship at this point, and that's ok. The reality is, if you aren't able to maintain your sobriety none of it will matter in the long run anyway, so you need to learn how to establish and practice being comfortable with boundaries first. Based on where you are in your recovery and your comfort level list some examples of boundaries you

would need to establish and communicate to someone you were in a relationship with, be specific.

_____

_____

_____

_____

_____

8. Part of being able to be in a loving relationship, is found in your ability to love yourself. At this point, can you honestly say, "I love myself"? Why or why not?

_____

_____

_____

_____

_____

9. If you answered, "No", to number 8, what specifically would you say is hindering you from loving yourself?

_____

_____

_____

10. What can you do in the future moving forward, to begin the process of loving yourself again?

Additional Workspace if Needed:

Section Ten

Giving Back

When looking at a life in recovery or any 12-step program after you are able to take an honest and through look at yourself and your defects of character to establish change in your life, you then have to look at how to maintain this in your life moving forward and avoid creating any new chaos or destruction. This is where giving back comes in. You need to look at your own behaviors and feelings daily (journaling helped me), but you also have to give to others what was so freely given to you. It never fails…. If I am irritable, discontent or in my head about things what works the best is to get out of myself. By helping someone else in need (either in or out of recovery), volunteering, listening to someone who just needs to talk, etc. I am able to gain perspective and my problems don't seem quite so big and loud anymore.

Early on I have had new comers ask me, "Roxanne, how is emptying ash trays or making a pot of coffee going to help me stay sober?". My answer is simply, "Because you are being of service to others and for this moment it's not about you and your troubles". Again, willingness and enthusiasm are not necessarily the same thing. Check your ego at the door. This is about being happy and fulfilled…..long term. Remember, the goal isn't just to GET SOBER, but learn how to STAY SOBER and live a LIFE OF RECOVERY! What are you good at? How can you give back? It takes thought after years of listening to negative internal dialogue to see your attributes and abilities clearly and how you are capable of helping others, and in turn helping yourself.

Section Ten Questions

1. What talents, skills, and/or gifts do you possess, which can enable you to be of service to others?

2. What, if any, negative self-talk are you still telling yourself, that would lead to you not feeling as though you could be of help to others?

3. What positive affirmations can you replace your negative self-talk with?

4. You heard in Roxanne's story about the fact that once she opened up about her past trauma, the best gift the person she was talking to at the moment could offer, was simply that of listening without judgment. Can you see the value in this? Why?

___

5. In what ways can you take a daily inventory and hold yourself accountable?

___

Additional Workspace if Needed:

___

Made in the USA
Columbia, SC
30 December 2024